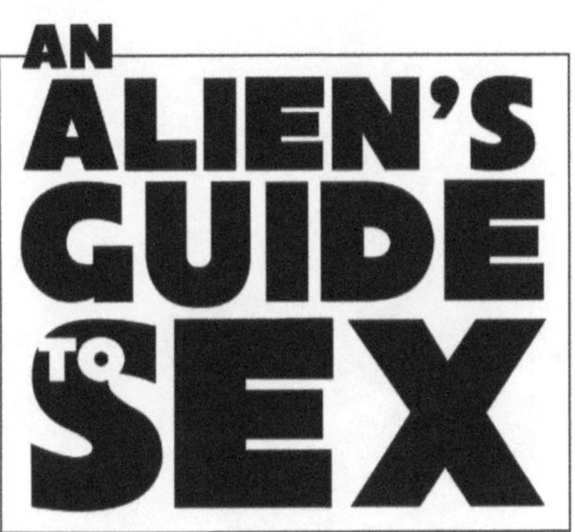

E.T.s & the ABCs of Human Sexuality

by

Bryce Morgan

ToC (re: E.T.s & the ABCs)

Why You Should Read this Book

Sex is important; very important. That's why you should read this book.

It shouldn't come as a surprise that most people would agree with that assessment. A vast majority of the planet's inhabitants would include sex on a *top ten* list entitled, "Good Things about Being Human". We like sex. But liking, even loving sex does not mean we understand sex. As was stated above, sex is important. Therefore, it's important we truly understand it.

When it comes to bodily urges, I suspect most people know sex is different than things like breathing and eating and 'taking a leak'. First of all, unlike those other bodily functions, you can survive without sex. Stop shaking your head, and think about it. You may not like the idea, but it's still true. Second, I believe all of us know sex is bigger than just the biology involved. Sure a good meal can seem like more than just putting 'gas' in your 'tank'. But please believe me, sex is bigger than that.

The purpose of this book is to show you that sex is even bigger than most of us think.

Why This Book Might Seem Too Alien for Some

I would argue that most people today have what we might call an *earthbound* view of sex. This limited perspective is clear from the way we obsess about sex, and exploit sex, and argue about sex, and look to sex for things sex cannot give us. To truly understand sex, we need a higher perspective, a view from above. What we need is *otherworldly* assistance.

If you picked up this book because you have an interest in risque science fiction, I hate to burst your bubble. Yes, this book is about sex and aliens, but not like you're thinking. This book is about two different *alien* perspectives, perspectives that may seem pretty alien to those with an 'earthbound' view of sex. But these alien perspectives can provide for us the very thing we need: otherworldly assistance; a view from above. Curious? Read on!

Sex and Satellite Navigation

Just like a satellite's view from above can provide navigation for bombers, boats, and Buicks, a higher perspective should guide our thinking when it comes to sex and sexuality (i.e., how we experience and express sexual desire). My aim in this book is to provide you with a kind of satellite navigation for sex by detailing both of these "alien perspectives". That's why there are two parts to this book.

Even though sex is bigger than the biological, it's critical we understand the biological. That's our focus in Part One. Yes, the first half of the book is full of fascinating facts you might feel you already know. But as you work through that information, I think you'll be challenged with some new ideas and perspectives. In Part Two, we'll connect sexuality and spirituality. If sex really is bigger than most of us think, then we need to acknowledge that life itself, that existence, is bigger than most of us think. Ever thought about how the meaning of sex is connected to the meaning of life? Yes, parts of this book might feel a little 'textbook-ish'. But sex is a powerful thing when it comes to the human heart. If we can find answers for those big questions about purpose, about love, about healing and happiness, about right and wrong, even about life and death, how could sex not be affected by such answers?

The two parts of this book are connected. You don't need to read or be persuaded by the second part in order to appreciate the first part, but you should. Why? Because sex is important, and even bigger than most of us think. If you want to find out how, keep reading. Otherworldly assistance is just ahead. In fact, if you listen carefully, you might just hear the strange hum of an approaching spacecraft.

Part One

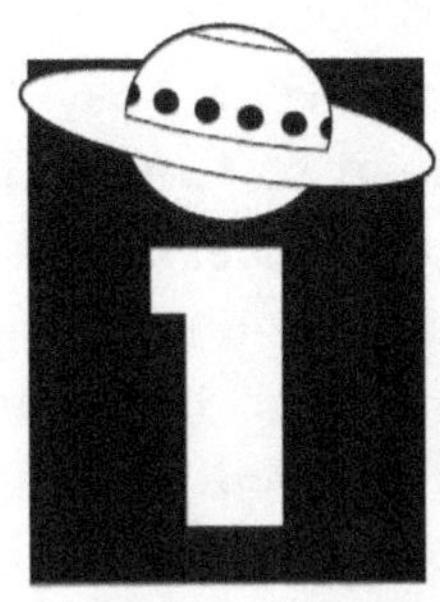

Alien Abductions

It was the twentieth century that gave us the phrase, "flying saucer". For decades after that phrase was introduced, movies and magazines were filled with intriguing illustrations of strange creatures from space visiting our world aboard these alien discs. But the popularity of these images was partly fueled by alleged sightings. Real people, from every walk of life, were claiming to have seen a saucer (or saucers) darting across the sky.

But in other cases, the claims were even stranger. Some had not only reported a sighting. Some had also reported an abduction... their own! You may be familiar with such claims: aliens from outer space abducting earthlings, taking them aboard their flying saucers, and then returning them to *terra firma* at some later time.

Now at this point, you must be scratching your head, thinking, "What does any of this have to do with sex?" Good question. Here's the connection:

many people who have reported being abducted have also described how they were analyzed by their alien abductors. And when I say "analyzed", I mean analyzed... from head to toe. And that includes the abductee's sex organs. Yikes!

Admittedly, that is a disturbing idea. But nevertheless, it is a useful idea in terms of that "satellite navigation" I described earlier. You see, even though there is very litte evidence that any of these alien abductions ever happened, the notion of this kind of awkward alien analysis is extremely believable. Of course alien visitors would want to study human beings. Of course they would want to understand us anatomically. We'd expect as much from any self-respecting, star-surfing space scientist.

Okay. Here's why this idea is so useful: the advantage of this hypothetical scenario is that these aliens would not be biased about sex. As asexual visitors from another world, the shadow of *subjectivity* would not darken their data. Their origins in a distant galaxy would give them a useful distance (a "view from above") when it comes to this often controversial topic. They would bring the very *objectivity* we often lack as human beings; as sexual beings.

Though we don't always think about it, objectivity is really, really important. To be objective is to be impartial. Think about why that's so important. If you were wrongly accused of murder, would you be okay with the judge and jury being the dead man's family? Uh... no. If your invention was vying for a billion dollar prize, would you be okay with the contest judges being the business partners of one of the other contestants? Uh... no. If you were a world class doctor, but suffering from a terrible and aggressive disease, should you be the one managing every decision of your medical care? Uh... no. Why "no" in all these cases? Because we all know how our feelings and relationships and loyalties and experiences can color our judgment as human beings. Wouldn't our thinking about sex also be affected by such things? To be fair, such subjective elements are not unimportant. But they should always come second (or else we will experience more and more friction, as our subjective world rubs up against objective reality—that is, what is really real outside of our thoughts and feelings and preferences). Again, this is why an alien analysis would be so helpful.

So the million dollar question becomes: what would this kind of alien analysis reveal about sex? If such creatures abducted five-hundred men and five-hundred women from across the globe (who, rest assured, would experience no discomfort and would have no memory of what happened), what would these intergalactic investigators conclude about human sexuality?

Wait. Look up in the sky! No, that isn't a hubcap soaring through the air. To use the old lingo, it's a *flying saucer*! And is that a door? Yes, a door is opening at the base of the saucer. And a ramp is being lowered. Let's climb aboard and discover what these aliens have discovered about us.

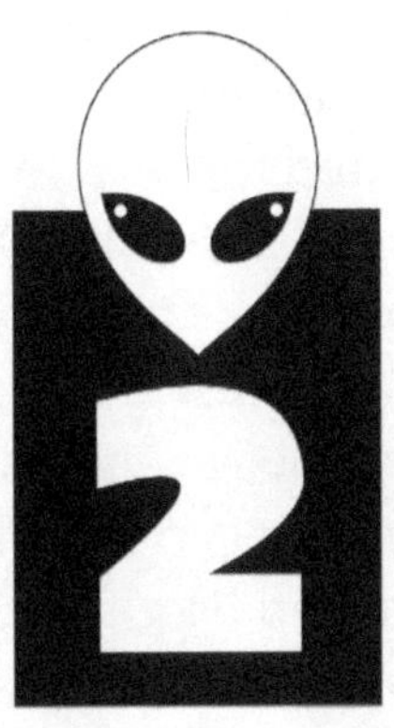

Four Scans

Surprisingly, these alien abductors are very hospitable. Who knew? They've guided us into a lab of some kind, and provided comfortable seats from which we can watch them carry out their research. And no, they are not using scalpels or lasers. They simply lay the unconscious human specimen on a long, smooth, silver table, then activate two floating probes that slowly scan the individual from head to toe, then toe to head. After a series of these flybys, data is transmitted to large screens placed all around the onboard lab. After the data appears on the screens, several aliens move from screen to screen, touching and sliding the surface in order to sort and interpret the information.

This whole process happens four times, with different scans alternating between inside and outside the specimen (scans one and three penetrating below the skin, even to the submicroscopic level). We also notice that each cycle is distinguished by lights of different colors pulsating on the floating probes (with the transmitted data also displayed in that same color on the lab's screens). After several hours of scanning and sorting, of computing and consulting, of modeling and musing over all one-thousand collected specimens, our alien hosts invite us to consider their data and their conclusions (warning: lots of 'science-y' talk ahead. Not super technical, but super interesting. I promise, thinking through it will be worth your time).

Scan #1: Inside

Looking deep inside their human specimens, these aliens would find the same binary reality (*binary* means characterized by two things) observable in the overwhelming majority of living organisms on our planet. Human beings, along with ninety-nine percent (!) of all animals, plants, fungi, and protists (tiny single-cell organisms) reproduce sexually. That means two distinct cells (called *gametes* or sex cells), from two distinct organisms, fuse in order to create a new organism. To clarify, "distinct" means these organisms belong to one of two types. They are either 'one' or the 'other'; 'this' or 'that'. And interestingly, it is that 'this/that' distinction that makes them compatible and life-creating.

In human beings, these space scientists would find that very same 'this/that' distinction in what human scientists have labeled *chromosomes*. Chromosomes are just long strands of DNA, the chemical code or genetic 'blueprint' that makes you *you*. We call the different sections of those long strands *genes*. Particular genes are a kind of code, one that directs particular molecules to make a particular protein. And those different proteins control different functions or create different cells, that then form the tissues that comprise a whole person. Try to wrap your mind around this: in the nucleus of every cell in their human specimens, these aliens would discover a complete set of chromosomes. You might think of it as your own DNA 'library'.

While some animals have more, and others less, humans have twenty-three pairs of chromosomes. These pairs are another reflection of that binary reality. Why? Because when those two gametes (sex cells) fused, half of those chromosome pairs came from 'this' and half came from 'that'. So in some sense, the new organism is a 'this/that'. But on the other hand, in light of that binary reality we talked about, this new organism, this new human being, must be either 'one' or the 'other'; either 'this' or 'that'. What makes the ultimate difference? That twenty-third pair of chromosomes (C-#23)!

The alien researchers would discover a 'this' kind of cell carries two of the same kind of C-#23, while a 'that' kind of cell carries a mixed pair. Human scientists describe these as "XX" and "XY" versions of a C-#23 pair. So how does this determine if the newly created organism is a 'this' or a 'that'? Unlike every other cell in the human body, gametes (sex cells) contain only twenty-three chromosomes (not the twenty-three *pairs* (i.e., forty-six total) described earlier). So in a 'that' gamete (remember, a 'half-the-chromosomes' cell), there will be either an "X" chromosome or a "Y" chromosome. If a 'that' with an "X" combines with a 'this', the new organism will be a 'this' (since a 'this' has only "X" chromosomes). If a 'that' with a "Y" combines with a 'this', the new organism will be a 'that' (because, at the most basic level, the "XY" version of C-#23 makes a 'that' a 'that')(don't feel bad if you have to read this paragraph again... I did).

Now at this point, these alien abductors may devise their own terminology to describe this binary reality, the 'this/that' nature of life on our planet. But what about us? What terminology do we use? Well, for a 'this' we simply use the word *female*, and for a 'that' the word *male*.

Scan #2: Outside

As these star-surfing scientists begin to show us results from their second scan, we quickly realize the focus is now on anatomy rather than microbiology.

As soon as their human specimens were collected (and probably even before, through their initial observations of our planet), it would have been abundantly clear to these researchers that the 'this' and 'that', or the *male* and *female* versions of our species have distinct anatomical differences. In fact, using their advanced technology, they could have predicted these differences simply based on our genetic information.

So the genetic differences inside us, the distinctions that helped us understand that binary nature of biological reality, are also evident on the outside. These differences are often referred to as *human* or *sexual dimorphism* (from the Greek language for "two forms"). While they would discover a number of anatomical differences (on average) in areas like muscle mass, lung capacity, heart size, height, and weight, these interstellar investigators would find the most significant differences between these "two forms" are related to the organs we call *genitals*.

Whatever letters, numbers, symbols, or weird clicking sounds our alien hosts would use to label these genitals, we generally refer to them as (in females) the *vagina* (and *vulva*) and (in males) the *penis* (and *scrotum*). Highly advanced scanning equipment and powerful computer modeling would allow these analyzing aliens to understand several aspects of the biological system to which these genitals belong. They would find...

1. *A Production System*

Our alien hosts would quickly discover that the differences in our genitals goes right back to the submicroscopic, binary reality highlighted in the first scan. For within the biological system to which the genitals belong, they would discover the means by which those fundamental gametes (sex cells) are actually produced. In males, this production takes place inside the scrotum, specifically in two small, round glands known as *testicles*. These testicles produce (millions everyday!) the male gamete, otherwise known as *sperm* (or *spermatozoa*). In females, this cell-producing gland is called an *ovary*. As with testicles in males, females each have two ovaries. And the female gamete produced by (or matured by) an ovary is called an *ovum* or *egg*.

2. A Delivery System

But these gametes cannot fuse unless they meet. And how can sex cells meet if they are inside the bodies of two distinct individuals? As these alien researchers would discover, the biological system to which our genitals belong also relies on a gamete delivery system. We refer to this transaction as *sexual intercourse*. While the tube-shaped male penis is normally flaccid (i.e., soft and hanging loosely), it has the ability to stiffen, as its sponge-like, inner tissue is filled with blood. At the same time, the vagina has the ability to secrete fluid, as it prepares for the penetration of the penis. These secretions both lubricate and reduce the acidity of the outer vagina, ensuring a safer passage for sperm (the male sex cell). After the male penis has penetrated the female vagina and is sufficiently stimulated, the male's genitals are able, through a series of muscular contractions, to forcefully expel (or *ejaculate*) semen (a whitish fluid that carries the sperm). In this way, tens of millions of sperm are delivered into the female reproductive system, in the hope that at least one will fuse with the female's ovum/egg.

3. *An Incentive System*

Finally, these alien scans would show that certain parts of both the male and female genitals include highly sensitive nerve endings. Before and during sexual intercourse, these physical areas, in response to stimulation, produce (in the brain) feelings of substantial physical pleasure. Moreover, such stimulation will finally lead to a climactic point of pleasure, typically referred to as *orgasm.* Significantly, orgasm is the point in males during which semen is expelled (or ejaculated) into the female. Therefore, our cosmic hosts, not surprisingly, have interpreted these pleasure responses as part of an incentive or reward system, a subsystem of the broader human reproductive system. Given that this system deals with the continuation of human life on our planet, the fact such behavior is incentivized comes as no surprise to our hosts.

Scan #3: Inside

As the color of the information on the alien screens changes, we realize we are now looking at the results of the third scan. Like the first, this scan also looked below the surface of the human body. But as our alien hosts explain, the focus this time is not on genes and gametes, but hormones. Hormones are signaling molecules, often called the body's 'chemical messengers'. They help regulate things like sleep, metabolism, respiration, and yes, even sex.

These curious space scientists would go on to show us how hormones are intimately involved in our human sexual system. First, hormones like *testosterone* and *estrogen* affect sexual motivation or drive (sometimes referred to as *libido*). Second, neurotransmitting hormones like *dopamine*, *norepineprhine*, and *serotonin* all work together to influence sexual attraction (dopamine affecting the so-called 'reward pathways' of the brain, thus linked with the incentive system discussed earlier). Finally hormones like *oxytocin* and *vasopressin*, produced in a part of the brain called the hypothalamus, affect attachment, promoting social/relational bonding. Interestingly, while oxytocin is produced at other times, under different circumstances, large quantities of the hormone are released during sex.

Scan #4: Outside

Before sharing their conclusions about human sexuality, our otherworldly guides point us to several screens containing information gathered from the fourth and final scan. As with the second scan, this final analysis pinpoints yet another outer, anatomical difference between the aliens' human specimens: the female breast.

Unlike her male counterpart, a female's breasts grow larger during puberty. Our friendly alien researchers go on to explain why. As children, both the male and female breast are composed of similar tissue. But as the female develops and that breast tissue grows, within each breast develops a network of ducts. And at the end of each duct is a cavity or sac known as an *alveolus*. It is here, in response to hormonal signals, that milk is produced in the mother's breast beginning in the eighteenth week of pregnancy. After a baby is born, that network of ducts then carries the mother's milk to the female's nipple, and finally to the feeding child.

Though it may seem like a strange question in our breast-obsessed culture, it's important to ask how the female breast is connected to the human sexual system. First, as our hosts have already indicated, the final development and unique purpose of the female breast is directly connected to the creation of a new organism through the fusing of the parents' sex cells. New baby, new changes in the breast! Second, the breasts (especially the nipples) contain (like the genitals) areas of sensitive nerve endings, that when stimulated can result in sexual pleasure. Third, there are hormonal connections to other parts of the human sexual system. Significantly, oxytocin is connected to the breast. This hormone, which as we learned, is released in large quantities during sex, is also released during breastfeeding. Oxytocin (as it works on an *alveolus*) not only makes breastfeeding physically possible, but it also (as was indicated earlier) promotes attachment/bonding between mother and child.

Having shared the results of their scans, the aliens are now staring at us with their unusually large, and unusually black eyes. Let's just say it's an awkward moment, on a number of levels.

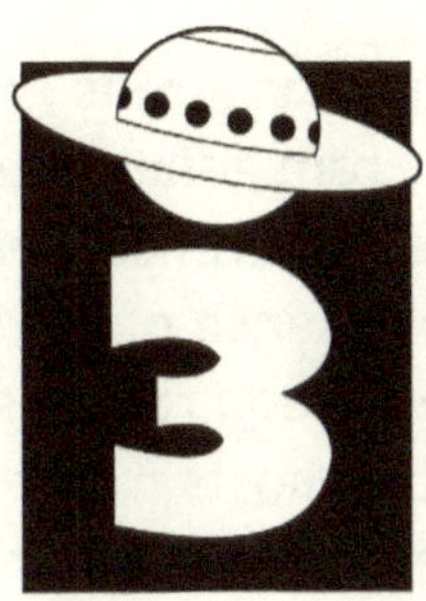

Their Conclusions

Now at this point, it would be understandable if some of us were having flashbacks of High School biology class. Some might say, "Don't we already know all this?" But remember, when it comes to sex, the issue is not ultimately a lack of data, but a lack of consensus on how to live in light of the data. And as was indicated earlier, these interstellar visitors (as non-human, asexual outsiders) have the kind of objectivity we need to sort out our *earthbound* ideas and conflicting assertions about sex and sexuality.

So what have our alien hosts concluded from their scans? They've concluded that sex and sexuality are rooted in and expressions of a biological system. And that biological system has been designed and functions in light of one goal: the creation and nurture of offspring. As we've seen, there are a number of important factors at work in this human sexual system, but all of them work together toward a reproductive end. Let's take a minute to consider some of those factors and our alien hosts' related conclusions:

The human sexual system is grounded in the reality of duality. From genetics to genitals, it is the distinctions, the differences between men and women that make sense of the human sexual system. The system requires this duality to work properly. Our alien hosts might explain it to us as a system focused on the 'other'. Not only does it absolutely require the 'other' (and in some sense, the 'otherness' of the 'other'), but amazingly, another 'other' is created when the system works optimally. And this other 'other' also reflects that initial duality, in that he or she is a genetic composite of the parents.

The human sexual system is all about connections. These alien analysts would also point out to us the importance of connection within the system. The obvious physical connection between the male and female genitals leads to the critical connection between their distinct sex cells (gametes). This then leads to another connection between the newly created embryo and the mother's body, a connection that will last until childbirth. But after childbirth, another connection is forged. Not only does the child connect physically to the mother's breast in order to feed, but through that connection, a relational or social connection is being formed as well. And in light of the similar hormonal response (remember *oxytocin*?), our hosts would be sure to point back to a similar connection between the sexual partners. It would be reasonable for them to propose that both of these bonds (between father and mother, and then mother and child) are important for the kind of nurture their *part me/part you* offspring will require.

The human sexual system utilizes human urges and feelings. In light of this alien data dump, we might chuckle, believing our extraterrestrial visitors have concluded sex is a sterile and clinical biological transaction. They would be sure to correct that judgment, reminding us of the hormonal and neurological (*neurology* concerns the body's nervous system) realities connected with sex. As our hosts pointed out earlier, these realities involve not only sexual motivation, but also sexual appeal and relational connection (i.e., appetite, attraction, and attachment). Think about it: how could the human sexual system function optimally if there was an indifference toward sex, or feelings of disgust over a suitable mate? And beyond the conception of a child, how well would the nurture of that child take place if there were only feelings of detachment and distance? These space scientists would certainly point out how the biological indicators confirm the place of feelings like passion and pleasure in the human sexual system.

Weaving these three aspects together in light of their main conclusion, these intergalactic investigators might say this about sex:

> *In light of the reality of human duality, the purpose of the human sexual system is to produce and nurture offspring by channeling passion and pleasure toward both a life-creating physical connection, and subsequently, a life-sustaining relational connection.*

Consider: what might it look like if this summary was the hub around which the spokes of our sexual perspective and practice revolved?

An Extremely Important Qualification

Having detailed for us the parts, processes, and purpose of the human sexual system, our galaxy-gliding hosts insist on showing us one more screen before we disembark. It is a massive screen filled with massive amounts of information. As they go on to reveal, this data represents an extremely important qualification to their carefully constructed conclusions.

What these aliens have been describing for us, in light of their scans, is not only the specifics of a biological system, but how that system runs *optimally*. As you may know, *optimal* means "best or most effective". When referring to something like a system, it means "operating exactly as it was designed to operate". But what this new screen displays are the ways, in their human specimens, in which the system is not operating optimally.

Like every biological system, every bodily system, the human sexual system can and does suffer from defects and disorders, abnormalities and conditions that cause it to operate *suboptimally*. For example, it could be that one of these alien abductees, one of their human specimens, has a sex chromosome abnormality. This means that instead of having a twenty-third chromosome pair that's "XX" (female) or "XY" (male), such an individual (who is still a *male* or *female*) might have "XXY", or "XYY", or even just an "X". While such abnormalities are very rare, they are also very real. The health effects of such a disorder can range from very minimal to very serious.

Similarly, the terms *hermaphrodite* or *intersex* can describe an individual characterized by one or more variations in terms of typical sexual development. Beyond chromosomal abnormalities, this kind of abnormality could result in a person having the reproductive hormones or genitals of the opposite sex, or a person having both kinds of genitals. Again, in terms of frequency, such genetic and developmental disorders are very rare. But of course the frequency does not make it any less difficult for those characterized by such disorders.

Other disorders of the human sexual system would include things like infertility and impotence (which can have many causes), or disorders related to hormones like testosterone and estrogen (with the body producing too little or too much). Of course, we could broaden our discussion of the *suboptimal* and include complications related to pregnancy, or disorders related to the brain and sexual appetite, attraction, or attachment.

But what does all of this mean for the aliens' assessment of the human sexual system? Do these deviations call their conclusions into question, or somehow 'muddy the waters'? Absolutely not. First, think about this: such variations would not be recognizable unless they were not what a researcher (or even non-researcher) would expect to see based on what is *typical*. Second, it is the *typical* that allows human or alien researchers to make sense of how the system operates, and how it operates optimally. Third, as stated before, there is no biological, no bodily system immune to defects and disorders. From the common cold to congenital birth defects, our bodies are prone to this kind of physical corruption. Ultimately, fourth, only what is *optimal* can help us make sense of and address these disorders.

With that in mind, consider if these aliens took pity on us and, in light of their advanced technology, sought to address our disorders and diseases. Maybe their very first step in doing this might be to equip us with a clear understanding of what is *optimal* and what is *suboptimal*. Why? Because if we are not anchored by what is *optimal* when it comes to these biological systems (including the human sexual system), then no matter what kind of technology we possessed, we would still struggle to both recognize and address what is *suboptimal*.

Suddenly, our session is cut short as the sunlight of a new day fills the room. Once again, a door at the

base of their spacecraft is opening. As we are escort-
ed off, we are reassured by two of the aliens that all
of their human specimens will be safely returned
home. We awkwardly shake their long three-fingered
hands, and slowly begin walking backwards through
a grassy meadow (not wanting to miss the craft's de-
parture). As the saucer rises up and darts out of
sight, we simply stare, attempting to process our
strange, strange journey.

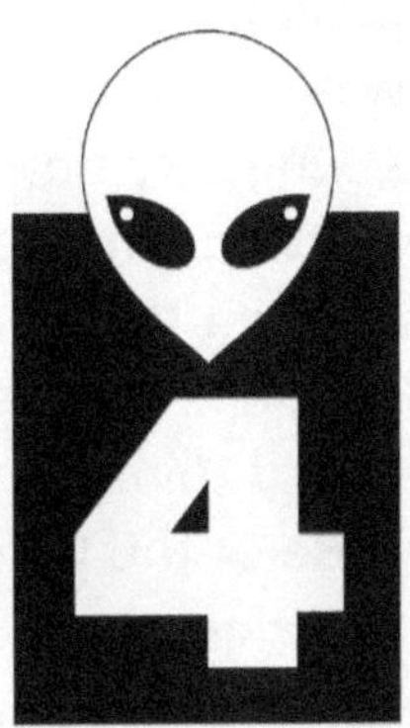

Our Conclusions

Most people would agree that the 'saucer sessions' described in the previous chapters could be accurately called "a strange, strange journey" for more than one reason. I'm guessing alien probes and conversations about sex with extraterrestrials would rank high on anyone's list of strange experiences. But for *earthbound* people like us, the alien assessment itself might be just that: *alien.*

Think about it: the conclusions of these space scientists might lead us to conceive of the human sexual system in terms of a series of connected realities (beginning with the act of sexual intercourse):

   Connection (physical)(intercourse)
→**Connection** (relational)(male/female)
→**Conception**
→**Connection** (physical (embryo))(mother/child)
→**Commitment** (male/female/child)
→**Connection** (physical*, relational)(mother/child)
→**Care**   [*Breastfeeding]

Obviously, these elements represent a broader perspective than the way many today think about sex. But remember, this summary flows out of an assessment of the whole system, an analysis of how every piece works together toward a biological purpose.

But do you find this alien assessment *alien*? Seriously. Take a second and think about how you would summarize the purpose of the human sexual system. How similar or how different would your summary be from that of the aliens? And how might your 'textbook' summary differ from the unspoken 'purpose statement' by which you live your life? Or if you largely agree with the aliens' assessment, and we look around at our culture, what do today's sexual banter and behavior reveal about our society's beliefs?

Think about this: if these alien abductors lingered and studied human society, just as they had studied human sexuality, they would almost certainly be scratching their smooth, overdeveloped craniums. Why? Because, in so many ways, our sexual behaviors would seem disconnected or detached from our sexual biology. Here are a few examples. These star surfers would observe...

Pleasure detached from purpose. Instead of ultimately serving as an incentive for reproduction, these space scientists would find us pursuing sexual pleasure as an end in itself. They might certainly grasp other ways sexual pleasure is important, but their ideas about a system focused on the 'other' would stand in stark contrast to our often selfish ideas about sexual stimulation. They would also discover...

Connection detached from conception. Even when we do crave intimate connection with another individual, our former hosts would observe how human society so often works to make sex more about romance and less about reproduction. Instead of that hormonal connection serving the important goal of bonding, then nurture, it too becomes an end in itself. As a result, our society utilizes its medical and scientific knowledge to neuter sex, using pills and procedures to keep the system from accomplishing its biological end. That's not to say our hosts would dismiss reasonable arguments for birth control. But they might question the extent to which we depict romance as a delight to be pursued and reproduction as a problem to be managed. Finally, these alien researchers would also observe...

Desire detached from duality. With pleasure detached from purpose, and connection detached from conception, it might not be surprising to these interstellar investigators that human beings have also disconnected sexual desire from the reality of our biological duality. If sex is turned into a self-serving enterprise, with one's own sexual stimulation being the only goal, then for some, at times, a sexual partner becomes unnecessary. Or a sexual partner could be someone of the same gender (normal biological urges being disconnected from the reality of duality). As long as sexual stimulation can be accomplished, even by alternative mechanisms, mechanisms that mimic the biological mechanisms of our human duality, many see no problem with this kind of 'disconnect'.

From adultery and masturbation, to 'friends with benefits' and pornography (in all of its 'colorful' and sometimes criminal manifestations), the only way these space scientists would be able to explain such behavior (behavior so disconnected from the purpose of this biological system) is by utilizing the language of defects and disorders.

Bigger than Biology

Of course, using words like "defect" and "disorder" when it comes to a person's sex life can feel uncomfortable (even judgmental), especially when we move beyond the physiological. When they do, the main reason these labels feel uncomfortable is that we believe sex is bigger than biology. In most cultures, sex and sexuality are also connected to things like love, acceptance, and personal identity. Moving beyond the aliens' assessment, most agree the factors that shape our sexuality are not limited to the biological. Our upbringing, peer pressure, our moral sensibilities, our religious beliefs, trauma we've endured, role models, social standards, all of these can and do shape our sexual perspectives and practices.

Where You Draw the Lines

But just as in the biological system, can't "defects" and "disorders" (i.e., deviations from the *optimal*) develop because of these less-quantifiable influences (i.e., upbringing, trauma, beliefs, etc.)? Almost all of us (with some disturbing exceptions) believe there are sexual beliefs and behavior that can and should be labeled as either *unhealthy*, or *immoral*, or *criminal*, or even *unconscionable*. Issues involving children, or animals, or harassment, or unfaithfulness, or self-harm, or public decency, or assault, or other forms of violence, are typically perspectives and practices around which people today draw sexual boundaries. So it's important to recognize that our clashing assertions about sex and sexuality are not, in most cases, at odds in terms of whether or not there are 'lines', but about where to draw those lines.

Based in the Biological

But if this is true, then why wouldn't our sexual standards (i.e., where we draw the lines) first be based on our biology? If this alien assessment taught us anything, it should have reminded us that sex is first and foremost a biological system. Think about it: this is proven by the simple fact that every single person reading these words exists only because of these biological realities of duality and reproduction. There's simply no way around that.

But instead of beginning with our biology, many today want to lay a foundation based on our feelings (whether our own feelings or the publicized preferences of others). Self, instead of cells, becomes our guiding light. Instead of looking to the *anatomy* of the self, we argue from the *autonomy* of the self when it comes to sexual standards.

The reason this is so concerning can be illustrated by thinking about another biological system: the human digestive system. From your teeth and your tongue, all the way down to your 'tailpipe', it almost goes without saying that the digestive system is absolutely vital. But like your sexual system, the digestive system is also bigger than biology. For humans, eating is more than just a biological transaction. Food and feasting can be (and are) also shaped by things like upbringing, culture, trauma, etc. For many, food preferences and practices help shape one's identity.

But as our medical knowledge has deepened, so too has our understanding of what is *optimal* when it comes to the digestive system. And that knowledge has made most of us aware of the fact that eating whatever we want, whenever we want, in whatever amount we want, will (sooner or later) have some very serious health consequences. If feeding is first based on feelings (e.g., having a 'sweet tooth', peer pressure, eating as escapism), eventually, I will suffer physically. But if my eating habits are first based in the biological reality of how my digestive system operates *optimally*, then I can assess and adjust my desires in light of what is healthy. What keeps us from applying the same reasoning to the human sexual system?

Consequences in Light of the Critical

So at this point, it might be a good idea to remind you of what I suggested at the outset: you may have an *earthbound* view of sex. After hearing the aliens' assessment and considering their conclusions, you may recognize that your ideas about sex and sexuality are rooted more in romance than reproduction; that your perspective is shaped more by your feelings than the facts of biology, or more by the media than the medical. But even still, you may respond with a genuine, "So what?" If *suboptimal* practices feel good and don't hurt anyone, some may ask, "Why does it matter?"

Based on what we've seen, it could be argued a *biologically consistent* view of sex matters for several reasons:

To begin with, the further we move away from the reality that sex is first about reproduction (and from related reproductive responsibilities), the more we threaten the healthiness (and eventually the existence) of the human species. For example, you can say you value trees (even being a self-described "tree hugger"), but if you are careless when it comes to seeds and soil and water, you are missing something critical about the biological reality of trees.

Second, expanding on that idea of human "healthiness", the more we make sex about *my* personal feelings and desires, the deeper we each sink into a kind of *me-centered* prison, one that threatens healthy relationships of all kinds (including between parents, and between parents and their offspring). This kind of orientation can result in not only emotional isolation, but even aggressive behavior, behavior driven by an unhealthy, self-grasping drive.

Third, the less clear we are on what is *optimal* and what is *suboptimal* when it comes to sex, the more difficult it will be to recognize and address the unhealthy factors that so often manifest themselves in our sexual deviations and disorders. For example, if we go back to the digestive system as a parallel, nutritional abuses can often be indicators of stress and anxiety. But only when we recognize such abuses as *suboptimal*, and are honest about their negative consequences, are we in a position to address the actual inner issues that drive things like overeating, and even 'under-eating' (e.g., *bulimia*). The same could be said about the human sexual system.

How We Truly Help

Okay. Let's say our perspective on sex has been genuinely persuaded by this alien analysis and assessment. If so, then how might we effectively address the *suboptimal*? We know when it comes to physiological disorders in our human sexual system, physicians can often prescribe a pill, or maybe perform a procedure (as with *impotence*, for example). But how do we address our common, but *suboptimal* beliefs and behaviors?

How do we help...

- The man whose sexual appetite is pulling him away from his wife and children?
- The woman who feels sexually attracted to other women?
- The teen who is escaping his difficult reality by immersing himself in pornography, sexual fantasy, and masturbation (subsequently, how do we help that same teen when, in his twenties, he is frustrated that real women are not like his pornographic 'dream girl')?
- A man or a woman who feels their gender identity is out of alignment with their chromosomal identity?
- A girl who confuses love with sex, or a man with an unhealthy interest in children, or a young couple feeling pressured because of their virginity, or a struggling, teenage survivor of molestation?

Clearly, in-depth answers to each of these questions is beyond the scope of this small book. But some general recommendations, some guidelines, might be helpful.

First, we work to avoid the extremes of either rejecting or relativizing. In both the past and present, there are some (apparently minimizing their own defects) who simply want to reproach, ridicule, and reject those struggling with sexually *suboptimal* feelings and behaviors. On the other hand, there are some who want to counter such negativity by declaring exactly the opposite, that is, that most of these feelings and behaviors are acceptable and natural (and in some cases, to be celebrated). But an accurate diagnosis (in light of our *alien* conclusions) should not be seen as incompatible with a gracious, respectful demeanor. We can and should talk about *unhealthiness* in terms of the human sexual system. But we can and should do so in a *healthy* way, with genuine care and concern for those in need.

Second, we 'set sail' for a better understanding, but without being 'anchor-less'. It is critically important we continue to investigate and dialogue about those things that can and do influence the human sexual system. But in our ongoing discussions and debates about 'nature versus nurture', we should not jettison the biological realities highlighted in the aliens' assessment. Instead (as was discussed earlier in "Based in the Biological"), we should hold onto what is most clear as we explore what is less clear.

Third, we apply this alien advice in our own struggles with the *suboptimal*. If we believe change is necessary in a world that is struggling sexually, then it's important we embody the very change we hope to see. What does this mean? It means that just as I am armed with the biological reality of how my digestive system operates *opti-*

mally, I can also assess and adjust my desires in light of how my sexual system operates *optimally*. Therefore, what might I need to unlearn and re-learn? What's to be received? What's to be rejected? What practical changes might be necessary to help that system function in a healthy way?

Fourth, we celebrate and make secure that which is *optimal*. Instead of glorifying depictions of sex and sexuality that deviate from the biological reality of the human sexual system, we should promote and protect healthy approaches, perspectives and practices that are consistent with things like connection, conception, commitment, and care.

I believe if we are serious about real answers and real help when it comes to sex and sexuality, we will discover there is helpful (though imperfect) advice to be found in what some might call *traditional wisdom*. Sometimes those who admirably want to 'advance' culturally believe progress only comes at the expense of traditional wisdom. But those often universally recognized beliefs about sex, reproduction, commitment, and nurturing children, those enduring basics of just being human, should be respected (especially since the biological realities highlighted by our *alien* assessment align with and affirm such truths). Yes, examples of this *wisdom* must still be sifted (for as in all things *human*, they too have been tainted). But with careful consideration (just as we've hopefully done in this assessment), I believe there is much to be gained when we 'stand on the shoulders' of past generations.

Wrapping Up

The alien spacecraft might have left our planet (maybe even our solar system), but you and I are still here. That means we have choices to make, choices informed by the truth. As sexual beings (that is, as creatures whose biological makeup includes a sexual system) we need to think carefully and consistently about how we use that system.

With that goal in mind, let's summarize what we've learned from the alien assessment detailed in this book, and our assessment of that assessment:

1. The male and female genitals, along with the female breasts, are part of a biological system, one which depends on the reality of our duality, and is designed to produce and nurture offspring.

2. Beyond the unseen cellular activity and obvious physical responses, sex also involves the hormonal responses evident in feelings like sexual appetite, attraction, and attachment.

3. But this biological system (like every other biological system) suffers from defects and disorders that cause the system to operate *suboptimally*.

4. Since sex and sexuality are broader than the biological, they are influenced by many other social, cultural, and emotional factors. These factors can either support the *optimal* operation of the human sexual system, or they can result in additional defects and disorders.

5. It is clear the human heart (each heart to some degree), and therefore human history, has been affected by these defects and disorders. And yet, since we often let feelings guide us (instead of the facts of biology), there is disagreement about the standards by which we assess the *suboptimal*.

6. Given the critical importance of this system (the mechanism by which you exist!), and therefore, the serious consequences of *unhealthiness* in this system, it is important each of us assess and adjust our thinking and living in light of what is *optimal*.

Consider for a minute all of the pain, suffering, confusion, and grief that has resulted (throughout human history) from our misplaced desires, our severed connections, our reflexive responses, our insensitive judgments, our rejected responsibilities, and our selfish rationales. While not dismissing other areas of human unhealthiness, certainly some of that harm could have been avoided had our sexual outlook been healthier, had it been *careful* in its formulation and *consistent* with our biology. Thus again, we see the importance of something like this alien (or *otherworldly*) assessment.

So stopping to catch our breath, it might be good to ask, "Does all of this make sense?" Has this alien perspective, has this "satellite navigation", has this "view from above" brought you to a new 'elevation' from which to see the 'big picture' of sex and human sexuality?

Even if you aren't persuaded (or *fully* persuaded), I hope I've challenged you to explore, and then eventually embrace, an outlook on sex/sexuality that makes sense of both the clear function of our biology and the common flaws of our beliefs and behavior.

Assertions about sex based simply on how people *feel* will eventually mire us in a slog of subjectivity. While feelings, preferences, experiences, and the like are certainly not unimportant, as I've argued, they must be tethered to the objective reality of the biological system to which our word "sex" is ultimately tethered.

Will a reformed/renewed outlook in light of our "saucer sessions" make all the difference? I don't believe it will. While a healthy outlook is the right foundation, it cannot ultimately change us in the way we need (which is change from *the inside out*). Real change is part of what I will explore in the second part of this book. But nevertheless, I hope this first half will both inform and inspire further thinking. I hope it will both challenge and change.

Part Two

Spiritual Aliens

At the outset I mentioned that the second half of this book would move us "from sexuality to spirituality". But what exactly does that mean? And why would such a step be important in a book about sex?

The Limits of the Physical

Though their assessment was incredibly helpful, the imaginary aliens we considered in the first half of the book could only tell us so much. Like scientists of the human persuasion, these aliens were able to detail the *how*, but not the broader *why*? Even though they could describe the workings of our bodies, they could not explain why our intricately beautiful bodies exist in the first place, and why they are the way they are (e.g., the reality of duality, the design of our sexual system, the presence of defects and disorders).

For many today, questions such as these seem unanswerable. Moreover, we often deem these issues as irrelevant to our everyday concerns. And yet, so many of our everyday concerns are driven by questions like...

- Why am I here, and is my life valuable?
- What does it mean to love and be loved?
- Why are my feelings of fulfillment so fleeting?
- How can I find healing and wholeness?
- What is truly right and wrong?
- Is death really the end?

Clearly, these are questions no scientist (whether star-surfing or earthbound) can answer. But nevertheless, they are critical questions. I think it's fair to say that our struggle to answer these questions is connected to the struggle we experience in so many areas of life, including the area of sexuality.

Spirituality Before Sexuality

Just as we needed the otherworldly perspective of our alien visitors to better understand (or reclaim an understanding of) the human sexual system, these more ultimate questions also require knowledge from above. But what we need revealed to us is far, far 'higher'... like *higher power* higher. You see, beyond *galactic* revelations, what we desperately need are *God's* revelations.

While in the minds of some God is a speculation, for this book he is a foundation. Let's think about why. The overwhelming majority of people on our planet believe in some kind of deity. Yes, some believe because they were taught or told to believe. But many believe because they recognize life is far bigger, far richer, far deeper, far more complex, far more ordered, far more beautiful, far more meaningful than random, natural processes could ever generate.

If *cause and effect* are indisputable features of reality, then tracing things all the way back, there must have been a *cause* for the *effect* we call the universe. That *uncaused cause* is God. Therefore, when it comes to life, God is like an author. If a book has *meaning*, it's because an author *meant* to communicate something. The same is true about life. Yes, you can try to make your life *meaningful*. But that doesn't mean you give it meaning in an ultimate sense. Only the Creator of life can give *meaning* to each and every life, for only he *meant* something when he created us (and the amazing universe in which we live).

Now, if you are unsure about the existence of God, there are many books and resources that can help you think carefully about this foundational idea (an encouragement: if you are someone who is skeptical about God, I'd ask you to keep an open mind, keep reading, and see whether these ideas make sense). As you might recall, this book is about sex. Therefore, it's important we 'connect the dots' when it comes to God and sex. How might we do that? By accepting the idea that God, that the Designer, meant something when he designed the human sexual system. Therefore, he is the one to whom we must go with our questions and disagreements about sex.

If God is in fact the Creator, then spirituality must always come before sexuality, that is, **the meaning of life must inform our ideas about the meaning of sex**. We would be mystified if we met a young auto mechanic who had every interest in the purpose of a transmission, but no interest in the purpose of a car. Admittedly, like the transmission in a car, our species won't get very far without sex. But if we are careless when it comes to overall purpose of a car, when it comes to the *operation* and intended *destination* of a vehicle, the relative importance of a transmission will quickly be put into perspective.

Answers from Ancient Wisdom

So where can I turn when it comes to the *operation* and *destination* of my life? Where might you look for this help from above, from beyond even the stars; in fact, from the One who made (!) the stars? The purpose of the second half of this book is to answer that question in light of the Christian faith. And that means looking to the ancient wisdom contained in those ancient writings known as the Old and New Testaments.

Okay. Obviously there are many religions and philosophies and systems of beliefs that claim to have knowledge from above, specifically, knowledge about the Creator and what he *meant* when he created us. But again, it's beyond the scope of this book to explore all of those belief systems. If you come across a book on Islam and sex, or Buddhism and sex, or sex and Sikhs, then you may want to consider those viewpoints. But I have written from a Christian perspective, not simply because I am interested in or prefer what that perspective reveals about sexual things, but because of what it reveals about *every-thing*.

Ask yourself this: does your *take* on the world make sense of the world? Does your view of reality correspond to the way things really are? The way we really are? Does your worldview address and make sense of not only human sexuality, but also those *ul-timate* questions (like the ones listed on page 40)? The premise behind this part of the book is that the ancient wisdom of the Christian faith provides just that: answers that really do make the best sense of life as it really is.

To be clear, this is not an affirmation of the supe-riority of Christians. It is an affirmation of the superi-ority of Christ, the *God-man* who revealed God to man in a superior way (remember, only the Author of life can help us with the meaning of life).

An *Alien's* Guide

One way in which the Christian perspective helps us make sense of human life is in the area of "defects" and "disorders"; those deviations that move us away from healthiness. And as you may remember, those defects, disorders, and deviations not only affect our bodies, but also our beliefs and behaviors. The Christian Scriptures have a name for this disordering, deviating force: *sin*.

For some, "sin" is an *antique-y* sounding word, one that simply refers to religious violations of one sort or another. But the Old and New Testaments describe sin as a 'worship disorder', as a 'what you live for', a 'what you love most' disorder. Instead of living for the One who made us for himself, all of us have chosen a *me-centered* path. And so we could say that **sin is living a me-centered life in a God-centered universe**. This orientation doesn't simply mean we fail to worship God as we should. It means we worship many things instead of God. We give our thoughts, our time, our affections, we give the trajectory of our lives over to things like pleasure, prestige, possessions, and power. To use the language of Scripture, we turn such things into *idols*. And if God is the greatest good imaginable, then this rejection, this rebellion, must represent the greatest offense imaginable, worthy of the greatest punishment imaginable. The word may sound "antique-y", but it's critical each of us grasp the reality and relevance of sin.

To be absolutely clear, we can and should distinguish between our personal choices and the broader effects of sin. Turning from our Creator has devastating consequences for us as creatures. When the human race decides to live *me-centered lives in a God-centered universe*, that discord with the Giver of life will inevitably affect the human race, body, soul, and spirit. So while our collective sin (what we might call *tainting* sin) does lead to physical degradation, disease, dysfunction, and ultimately death within the human race, it doesn't mean every physical defect, disorder, and deviation is the result of a specific person's specific sin (what we might call *tempting* sin).

But in regard to our personal choices (that *tempting* sin), if sin really is a 'worship disorder', a 'what you live for', a 'what you love most' disorder, what does that mean in terms of sex? First, it helps us understand the power of our sexual sin. As an expression of a 'worship disorder', sexual sin grips our whole heart. It wraps itself around and warps our sense of identity and purpose. Second, this idea of sin as a 'worship disorder' helps us understand the pervasiveness of our sexual defects, disorders, and deviations. There is no individual and no culture unaffected by this *me-centered*, God-neglecting orientation. While these defects, disorders, and deviations have affected different cultures in different ways, there is no society, past or present, that has not dealt with, even delighted in, sexual beliefs and behavior at odds with the purpose of the human sexual system.

Now think for just a minute about what that would mean for anyone who attempted to live a *God-centered* (instead of a *me-centered*) life, and specifically in this area of sexual beliefs and behaviors. Two thousand years ago, a man named Peter wrote to encourage his readers to do this very thing:

Beloved, I urge you as aliens and strangers to abstain from fleshly lusts which wage war against the soul. (I Peter 2:11)(NASB)

So the saucer-riding, star-surfing variety are not the only kind of *aliens* we need to consider. Like foreigners living in a land that's not their own, those who follow Jesus Christ can provide a very different perspective on sex and sexuality; what we might call an 'outsiders' perspective. But again, this does not come from them. It comes from the One they follow; the One who stepped *inside* humanity from *outside* the world, in order to save the world. It is this other *alien* perspective that we'll explore in the next chapter. As we do, let's think very carefully about how that perspective lines up with our original alien assessment.

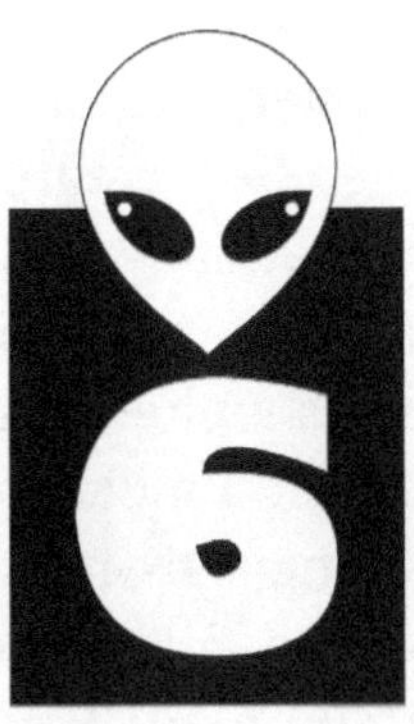

The Designer's Design

If they had the chance, I believe our saucer-surfing scientists would be extremely eager to talk about the human sexual system with the designer of that system. Even though they possess knowledge and technological know-how that far surpass our own, they would surely recognize that God's creative efforts were on a whole other level. As the ancient Hebrew king, David, declared: "I will praise you because I have been remarkably and wondrously made." (Psalm 139:14a)(CSB)

But what about us? Are we also eager to hear from the divine Designer? To learn about the meaning of sex from the One who *meant* something when he made something like sex? Let's do this by turning to the earliest pages of the Old Testament.

Genesis and Our Genesis

The opening chapters of the ancient Jewish book of Genesis are an account of how God created the universe. But not surprisingly, this account is focused on the origin of our planet, rather than the 'bazillion' other heavenly bodies God created. To be clear, the Genesis account of creation was not first recorded by or for modern journalists and scientists. Instead, it was given to farmers, shepherds, and craftsmen who lived in the Middle East almost four thousand years ago. So instead of being a six-hundred volume set of massive books chocked full of scientific data, this record is a simple summary (composed of around thirteen hundred words) covering two short chapters (Genesis 1 and 2) at the beginning of the biblical record.

But even though this account was written for *ancients*, it is not in any way less true for *moderns* like us. Why? Because these chapters are about every human being and why we exist. For example, after the creation of things like stars, starfish, and starlings, Genesis 1:26 tells us...

> *Then God said, "Let us make man in our image, after our likeness. And let them have dominion over the fish of the sea and over the birds of the heavens and over the livestock and over all the earth and over every creeping thing that creeps on the earth."*

If you read through the first twenty-five verses of Genesis 1, what is striking about the twenty-sixth verse is that, of all the living creatures on planet Earth, only humanity is said to be made in God's image (to be clear, the "our" used by God in this verse is most likely a kind of 'royal *we*', something a king might say when making a decree). But what does it mean that we are made in God's image?

From the 'classics' to cartoons, artists have often depicted God as some kind of glorified man (usually as an old guy with a flowing white beard). But the rest of the Old Testament confirms that God is no man. Genesis 1:26 tells us that being made in God's image is not connected to how we *look* (and thus, how God looks), but our calling to *look after* this planet we call home. This is clear from the fact that terms like "image" and "likeness" are immediately followed by a call to "dominion" (i.e., to rule or reign over). So what distinguishes human beings from every other creature is that we were created and equipped for leadership, just as God is the highest Leader (of course, this kind of leadership requires us to possess many other qualities that distinguish us from every other living creature on the planet, including the capacity to know God).

But notice what the next verse in Genesis 1 reveals about this divine image...

So God created man in his own image, in the image of God he created him; male and female he created them. (Genesis 1:27)

Did you notice the last part of verse 27 points out how the word "man" is being used in the first part of the verse? The writer is speaking about man in the sense of "*man*kind" or "hu-*man*-ity". This is clear from the fact that God created "man" in two distinct versions: "male and female". But remember, it is "man" who was created in God's image, that is, humanity was made in his likeness. Why is it important to point that out? Because it is in our duality that we reflect the image of the One who made us (notably, that reflection includes the capacity to love as God loves, with a self-giving, other-directed love).

Just as our alien hosts observed, beginning with our chromosomes, there is a fundamental reality of duality when it comes to humanity. And that duality must also be connected to our destiny, a destiny (as we saw) defined by "dominion" (v. 26). So reigning over God's creation, as creatures appointed by God himself, requires both *maleness* and *femaleness*. But how and why? It's that question that drives us back to the main topic of this book: sex.

Multiply Via Monogamy

Our linkedness in his likeness is explained in the very next verse of Genesis 1. In verse 28 we read...

> *And God blessed them. And God said to them, "Be fruitful and multiply and fill the earth and subdue it, and have dominion over the fish of the sea and over the birds of the heavens and over every living thing that moves on the earth."*

To reign over the planet, humanity must cover the planet. Faithful management as God's image-bearers must be a locally-sourced commodity. But to be local leaders, humanity must be larger.

Now wait. When "God created man [humans] in his own image", how many did he make? Well, the next chapter of Genesis answers that question. We read in chapter 2, verse 7 that...

...the LORD God formed the man of dust from the ground and breathed into his nostrils the breath of life, and the man became a living creature.

A little further into that same chapter, after "the man" finds no suitable companion among the animals, we read about an interesting account (in 2:21, 22) of divine anesthesia and surgery...

So the LORD God caused a deep sleep to fall upon the man, and while he slept took one of his ribs and closed up its place with flesh. And the rib that the LORD God had taken from the man he made into a woman and brought her to the man.

So the answer to our question is *two*... when God first created human beings, he made two of them; "male and female", just as 1:27 described. But as was stated earlier, to be local leaders, humanity must be larger. This means the first man and the first woman needed to do the very thing God told them to do: "be fruitful and multiply and fill the earth".

While all of this is vitally important, it is no over-statement to say that what we read next in Genesis 2 is truly central when it comes to making sense of sex. The writer of Genesis emphasizes the fact that God taking the first woman *out of* the first man, and then taking the first woman *to* the first man, established a divine precedent, a kind of God-provided pattern for every other couple to come. This is how the writer expresses it...

Therefore a man shall leave his father and his mother and hold fast to his wife, and they shall become one flesh. (2:24)

When it comes to understanding the Designer's design, when it comes to understanding what the Old and New Testaments teach about sex, the key is found in the final phrase of verse 24: "one flesh". In light of the context, the first readers of Genesis would have understood that phrase to be a reference to both sex and marriage.

As is clear in the verse, ancient marriage customs are certainly in view: a man leaving his parents' home in order to cling to "his wife" and establish their own home. Therefore, a man leaves his "flesh and blood" in order to become "one flesh" with his wife. That's a statement about family or kinship. But it's also a statement about sex. Just as the first woman was taken *out of* the first man, marriage involves a man going *into* a woman, thus reconnecting the two parts of humanity. And if we keep the context in mind, all of this is connected to God's original mandate:

"Be fruitful and multiply and fill the earth and subdue it..." (1:28)

Jesus on "One Flesh"

The New Testament also speaks about this "one flesh" union and even fleshes out (pun intended) the implications of this key concept. This is best seen in the words of Jesus, in the very first book of the New Testament. When asked by certain Jewish leaders about acceptable grounds for divorce, Jesus answered,

> *"Have you not read that he who created them from the beginning made them male and female, and said, 'Therefore a man shall leave his father and his mother and hold fast to his wife, and the two shall become one flesh'? So they are no longer two but one flesh. What therefore God has joined together, let not man separate."* (Matthew 19:4-6)

While their question was posed in light of the fifth book of the Jewish Scriptures (i.e., Deuteronomy, specifically 24:1-4), Jesus took these leaders back to the first book of the Jewish Scriptures (i.e., Genesis). It was in the creation account that these teachers would find their answer, specifically in the "one flesh" verse we just highlighted, Genesis 2:24.

Take a second to read Jesus' words one more time. Do you see what he's telling us about this "one flesh" union? First he affirms both the reality and utility of humanity's duality ("he...made them male and female"). Then there's a "therefore". Then Jesus quotes the remainder of Genesis 2:24. Finally, he addresses their original question. "Divorce?" Jesus seems to ask, "No, you should not separate what 'God has joined together'". Just like the writer of Genesis, Jesus understood the precedent and pattern of that very first God-forged union. Therefore, every marriage, every union like that first union, where male and female are one again, is astonishingly, an act of God.

Like the author of Genesis, the Apostle Paul, an early Christian leader, also understood the phrase "one flesh" to refer to both a physical union (read for example, I Corinthians 6:16) and a relational union, that is, to the marriage bond God himself creates. Paul understood what Jesus taught when he said, "So they are no longer two but one flesh." (Matthew 19:6a) In light of this, the Apostle also helps us understand additional implications of this "one flesh" union. He writes in Ephesians 5:28-31...

> *In the same way husbands should love their wives as their own bodies. He who loves his wife loves himself. For no one ever hated his own flesh, but nourishes and cherishes it, just as Christ does the church, because we are members of his body. "Therefore a man shall leave his father and mother and hold fast to his wife, and the two shall become one flesh."*

(Surprise, surprise...it's Genesis 2:24 again!)

Paul makes it clear that God's design for sex and marriage involves a context in which words like "love", "nourish", and "cherish" are defining characteristics; a context in which a oneness of bodies is reflected in a oneness of hearts and minds.

Conclusion and Comparison

So as we've seen, from Genesis to Jesus, and from Jesus to Paul, both the importance and implications of the "one flesh" union are set forth in the Old and New Testaments. But I think it's important to explicitly 'connect the dots'. Consider the following conclusions about sex in light of what we've learned regarding the Designer's design:

1. Unlike the other creatures God created in the beginning, Genesis 1 tells us humanity was made "in the image of God" (v. 27). We learned that this does not refer to our *appearance*, but to our *appointment* as 'deputy rulers' over the planet (vs. 26, 28).

2. We also learned that humanity was created in two versions, "male and female" (Genesis 1:27). Since mankind is said to be made in God's image, both *maleness* and *femaleness* must complement one another in reflecting, through our reign, the character of the One who made and reigns over all things.

3. But there is even more utility to our duality. To properly manage the planet, humanity must cover the planet as God's image-bear-

ers, uniquely reflecting the Creator's goodness throughout his creation. Of course, to do this, mankind must be able to multiply. Thus, God created the human sexual system. Therefore God's design makes sense of and makes possible his decree: "Be fruitful and multiply and fill the earth and subdue it..." (Genesis 1:28).

4. Finally, we learned that God also created a relational union to mirror the physical union (both described with that phrase from Genesis 2:24, "one flesh"). Why this relational union? Because his design was focused not simply on the production of children, but also on their nurture. Not only is the vital commitment between a father and mother meant to provide vital stability for the formation of their family, but each gender provides a unique and necessary influence in terms of a child's nurture. As the writer of Genesis makes clear (and Jesus confirms), this relational union is what we call (and most cultures have called) *marriage*.

In light of these conclusions, here's something to consider: though this broad description can sound dispassionate, it is in no way contrary to the passions and pleasures of sex. But when the Scriptures commend sexual pleasure, they do so within the context of marriage (cf. Proverbs 5:15-19). Only within marriage is sexual pleasure purposeful in accordance with God's design. It not only nurtures the bond between husband and wife, but in so doing, it fortifies a family's foundation (regardless of that family's stage of life). Could we therefore say that sex is about more than reproduction? In one sense, yes. Physical and emotional intimacy should go hand in hand, and are part of God's good design for sex in marriage. But pleasure and reproduction, as well as closeness and nurture are all part of the same system; that system designed by the Designer of all things. So we could say that even when defects and disorders mar the system, these aspects remain important. For example, a couple struggling with infertility still benefits from the emotional intimacy of sexual connection. That strengthened relational bond is valuable for many reasons, even when there are no children in the home.

Something else to consider: in light of this discussion about God's design for sex and marriage, it's important to point out that the Christian Scriptures recognize, and even (in one sense) recommend, the benefits of singleness. In an ancient letter we call First Corinthians, Paul wrote, "I wish that all were as I myself am" (7:7)(that is, single). Why singleness? Paul went on to tell his readers, "those who marry will have worldly troubles, and I would spare you that." (7:28) Was Paul badmouthing God's good design for marriage? Absolutely not! Paul knew not everyone was called to a life of singleness (cf. 7:7). In addressing singleness, he was writing from the perspective of Christian ministry, and what is practically preferable. This is why he goes on to explain:

> *I want you to be free from anxieties. The unmarried man is anxious [concerned] about the things of the Lord, how to please the Lord. [33] But the married man is anxious about worldly things, how to please his wife, [34] and his interests are divided... [35] I say this for your own benefit, not to lay any restraint upon you, but to promote good order and to secure your undivided devotion to the Lord.* (7:32-35)

Thus in light of knowing and serving God, chaste singleness (whether for a season or for a lifetime) also has an important place in God's design.

So stop and catch your breath again. When you do, think about two things in light of the Designer's design:

First, consider how big this understanding of sex really is. It goes from the cradle to the Creation (i.e., from the formation of a human baby to the formation of human society). It is both global and God-ward, parent-focused and planet-focused. It includes both the physical and relational connections. It focuses on responsibility and purpose, without sacrificing romance and pleasure. Unlike so much modern thinking (which is decidedly *me-centered*), the Designer's design, as revealed in the pages of Scripture, is both profoundly personal and personally profound. Though many today, for all intents and purposes, 'worship' sex, only God's *alien* can truly appreciate the sacredness of both sex and marriage, two strands designed by the Designer to be integrally intertwined. In light of this, it's no wonder that one New Testament author urges his readers to, "Let marriage be held in honor among all..." (Hebrews 13:4a)

Second, consider how this vision for sexuality compares to what our alien hosts discovered about the human sexual system. Point for point, what God has revealed corresponds to what their saucer scans revealed about connection, conception, commitment, and care. What does that mean? It means there are very good reasons to anchor our understanding of sex in what God has revealed in Scripture, since what God has revealed best corresponds to what is objectively true about the human sexual system.

Of course, many today would take issue with that claim. But as we will see in the next chapter, objections to this conclusion are usually rooted in estimations that attempt to make the *suboptimal* optimal, perspectives that downplay the defects, disorders, and deviations that, in one way or another, characterize everyone one of us and every part of our lives (including our sexuality). But as we've seen, God is not silent.

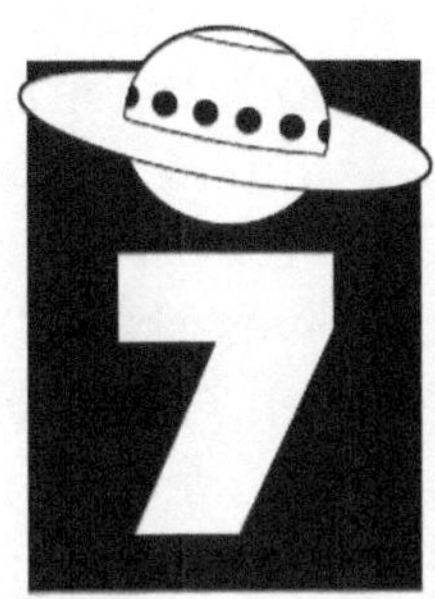

Perspective & Practice

Ever seen those old photos or movies of astronauts on a 'spacewalk'? While our alien abductors might have a more advanced way of moving outside their saucer, those first human astronauts utilized at least three things: 1) a sealed spacesuit, 2) a small propellant device to get around, and 3) a tether (i.e., a hose that supplied oxygen to the astronaut and kept him connected to his capsule).

While the first item was essential, the second was more of a luxury. But more important than either of these was item number three. Think about it: the freedom of floating in space, high above the Earth, was only possible because of that tether. Exhilaration by way of limitation. Restriction that allowed incomparable exploration. Was a spacewalk possible without such a tether? Of course... if your idea of a good time is floating off, alone, into the cold darkness of our solar system.

Did you know tethers are also important for us non-astronauts? Limits. Restrictions. Boundaries. In spite of what many in our society advocate, all of these are critical for both maintaining and enjoying life. But is that how you think about sex?

Perspective informs practice. And so, for many today who believe our lives should be guided by our own desires, rather than God's desire for our lives, sexual expression has very few boundaries. When men and women, and young men and young women, hold to the "autonomy of the self" in all matters, we see a distortion of God's design for sex: pleasure detached from purpose, connection detached from conception, and desire detached from duality.

But sexual standards rooted only in what 'feels good' or 'feels right' to a particular individual can never truly be fixed or firm. When such subjective standards are not tethered to anything objective (like our biology), sexual discipline, sexual boundaries, and sexual accountability become slippery concepts for which to advocate. Following such a path, eventually, any prescribed restriction on one's sexual impulses will be questioned... and then resisted. As long as *self* informs our society's standards, we will find ourselves on shifting sands. The boundary lines will continue to be redrawn, even in places we deem unthinkable today.

The Jewish Scriptures (in Proverbs) speak about the dangers of this *me-centered* perspective...

There is a way that seems right to a man, but its end is the way to death. (14:12, 16:25)

Everything Outside the Circle

But what if God's perspective, and not *self*, informed our practice? In light of the 'big picture', the broad *cradle to Creation* perspective presented in the previous chapter, I think we can affirm one clear, core principle when it comes to healthy sexual practice:

Sexual desires and delights were designed for the commitment-clad, life-nurturing, one man-one woman context of marriage.

The "one flesh" emphasis of the Old and New Testaments provides the most important *reference point* when it comes to sexual practice. This means the marriage union between a man and woman represents a kind of *circle of safety* when it comes to sex. Therefore, there are very difficult emotional, physical, relational, societal, and spiritual consequences when we take sex outside God's *circle of safety*, marriage.

But as we've seen, the Jewish and Christian Scriptures describe that tendency as our default. As sinners, as those marked by a deeply ingrained 'worship disorder', we are prone to wander outside that circle. Defects and disorders are the norm in our broken world. Consequently, as long as we are not tethered to God's design when it comes to sex, we will continue to struggle identifying what is healthy and unhealthy, what is optimal and suboptimal, what is right and wrong.

This is why it is critical for us to start with God's reference point for sex: *the commitment-clad, life-nurturing, one man-one woman context of marriage.* Let's think for a few minutes about how that perspective should shape our practice.

Today's FAQs About Sex

God's guidance begins with his reference point: marriage. But the Jewish and Christian Scriptures go on to give us what we, in light of our culture, might call an *alien's guide to sex.* So how can God's countercultural wisdom guide us when it comes to our sexual beliefs and behaviors? Below are some common areas of concern, and often, confusion. So much more could be said about any one of these topics. But a very brief overview will have to suffice. For example, consider...

Marriage: If marriage is God's garden, the good soil in which our sexual desires can truly flourish, then it's important we think about marriage according to what he's revealed. Marriage is not simply the next chapter in a fairy tale romance, or some contractual obligation in effect as long as two people stay 'in love'. The Scriptures teach us that marriage should be a selfless commitment, inspired by Jesus' own love for his people (cf. Ephesians 5:25-27). This selflessness should be expressed in every area, including the bedroom. The Apostle Paul expressed this very point in a chapter we looked at earlier, First Corinthians, chapter 7. This is verses 3-4...

The husband should fulfill his marital duty to his wife, and likewise the wife to her husband. The wife does not have authority over her own body but yields it to her husband. In the same way, the husband does not have authority over his own body but yields it to his wife. (NIV)

This is a far cry from the kind of ethic that puts my sexual satisfaction above everything else. Of course, this self-giving mindset is bigger than sex. This other-focused love not only helps couples weather the inevitable struggles of life, but also to create a nurturing environment in which children can similarly flourish. Therefore, while divorce will always be present in a *me-centered* world (and in some cases, unavoidable), it is a deviation from God's ideal for sex (i.e., connection, conception, *commitment*).

Premarital Sex: When it comes to sex, our culture often thinks more about recreation and less about procreation. Many today tell us that because sexual urges are natural (i.e., bodily) urges, we should satisfy them when and however we see fit (as long as no one else is 'hurt' by our actions). This has led many to engage in sexual activity *untethered* from marriage. The Christian leader Paul understood the reality of these urges, but gave very different advice in First Corinthians...

But because of the temptation to sexual immorality, each man should have his own wife and each woman her own husband. (7:2)

In pointing his readers to marriage, Paul was reminding them about the goodness of God's design, that marriage is a reality worth waiting for. In contrast, when sexual union is disconnected from the commitment-clad union of marriage, when there is no bond beyond intercourse, there will always be an emotional toll. And if a child is conceived in the process, he or she may not know God's ideal: the incomparable influence of the interwoven lives of his or her mother and father; of the daily influence of the dynamic duality of God's image bearers.

Adultery: There's a reason adultery is addressed in number seven of what the Hebrew Scriptures call the "ten words" (most people know them as the "Ten Commandments"). Sexual unfaithfulness strikes at the very heart of God's design. Even when the sexual ethics of a culture are more *me-centered* than *God-centered*, oftentimes, there is still a recognition that adultery is a painful betrayal. That recognition of betrayal should point us back to the importance of one's marital vows and the marriage bond itself. Even when couples struggle with intimacy, a wife should never tolerate a husband's sexual digressions. Neither should a husband tolerate his wife's emotional entanglements with other men (and vice versa in terms of physical and emotional unfaithfulness). Adultery should never be justified or minimized. Instead, a husband and wife must work hard to guard their hearts, and fight to live in and live out the unity that is theirs through marriage.

Masturbation (and Fantasizing): In Part One, we looked at the fact that many people today want to separate sex from the reality of our duality (i.e., maleness and femaleness), focusing on sexual pleasure apart from the purpose of the human sexual system. One way in which we do this is masturbation. No doubt, many will scoff at the idea that masturbation is wrong, since, as they believe, the practice doesn't hurt anyone and provides a needed sexual release. But how can this kind of self-stimulation not reinforce the idea that sex is primarily about my own sexual pleasure? And if sexual arousal requires fantasizing (i.e., mentally entertaining imaginary sexual partners and/or scenarios), how could such behavior not turn someone more and more inward, so that they begin to prefer lies to the truth. How could such behavior help and not hinder the self-giving call of God's sexual design within marriage? Jesus gave us a right estimation of such behavior when he declared...

"You have heard that it was said, 'You shall not commit adultery.' But I say to you that everyone who looks at a woman with lustful intent has already committed adultery with her in his heart. If your right eye causes you to sin, tear it out and throw it away. For it is better that you lose one of your members than that your whole body be thrown into hell. And if your right hand causes you to sin, cut it off and throw it away. For it is better that you lose one of your members than that your whole body go into hell." (Matthew 5:27-30)

Notice how Jesus first connects adultery with lust-filled thoughts, then, apparently, lust with masturbation ("right eye" to "right hand"). His charge is clear: radically reject those beliefs and behaviors, those attitudes and appetites, that do not align with God's own *true-to-his-word* (promise keeping) nature and his commitment-clad, other-focused design for sex.

Pornography (and our "Sexy"-Saturated Culture): Whether married or unmarried, God calls us to direct our sexual desires to our (current or future) spouse. In contrast, pornographic material invites you to direct your desires toward a sexual fantasy. Yes, the models in a pornographic image or video may be real, but they are peddling lies about sex, the very lies our culture wants to believe: pleasure detached from purpose, connection detached from conception, and desire detached from duality. Pornography simply feeds the same self-focused orientation mentioned in reference to masturbation. It trains us to prefer fantasy over reality, which in turn warps our sexual expectations. It turns human beings into nothing more than human bodies, and human bodies into nothing more than vehicles for self-gratification. Take a minute to think about the toll this takes on marriage. If God's design for lovers is a physical, emotional, and relational union, how could this union not be hurt by the warped expectations pornography produces?

Of course, pornography is not the only mass medium or mechanism designed to be sexually stimulating. While most would not label them pornographic, television is filled with images that are definitely sexual or sensual. We could add to this magazines, romance novels, billboards, sporting events, comic books, and even video games that feel compelled to 'spice it up' with shirtless men and busty women. Moreover, so much of our popular music is also sexually saturated. Similarly, there are styles of dress, fashion that aims for "sexy", encouraging their wearers to proudly 'show some skin'. While every culture has different standards in terms of what is appropriate and inappropriate, of what is modest and what is immodest, every culture also knows that 'sex sells'. No culture is without this taint.

But the man or woman who is looking to God's *reference point* for sex, who is tethered by the truth about God's design, will attempt to steer clear of such things. Acknowledging the many variables involved in people's perceptions and preferences, he or she will, nevertheless, be sensitive to the sexual weaknesses of others, as well as to his or her own weaknesses. What does that mean practically? It means these weaknesses should affect how we look (i.e., our garb) and how we look (i.e., our gaze). The *alien's* interest in stimulating or being stimulated will be fixed on the reality of one's (current or future) spouse, not on the empty fantasies of a *me-centered* culture.

Homosexuality (and Gender Confusion): So much of what we've seen thus far in terms of practice could be summed up as "misdirected urges". As our intergalactic investigators described for us, sexual attraction and appetite are important parts of the human sexual system. Can you imagine a system in which the means of multiplying is broadly considered horrifying? Or one in which union is just plain uninteresting? But as we've seen in this study, and as we know from our daily news, these desires can also be misdirected.

Consider homosexuality as yet another example. Not all homosexual behavior is driven by the same factors. But in many cases, homosexuality is one more expression of these misdirected urges. In a world in which each of us is affected in some way by the defects, disorders, and deviations of our bodies and minds, of both biological systems, as well as beliefs and behavior, it should not be surprising that some deal with an attraction toward and sexual appetite for someone of the same gender. For many, those feelings have been present for as long as they can remember.

But even when an individual does not choose the feelings/desires they experience, they can choose what to do with those feelings (generally, we expect such sexual responsibility when it comes to our urges). If our alien assessment is correct, then homosexuality is clearly out of step with the purpose of the human sexual system. Like many other expressions of human sexuality in this fallen world, it is *suboptimal* in terms of God's design for merger and multiplication.

But homosexuality is not alone in terms of duality-disordering challenges. Some individuals experience gender confusion, not just in terms of sexual attraction and appetite, but also in terms of their essential identity. Though biologically male or female, a number of people feel as if their true gender identity does not match their physiology. While these feelings must be extremely difficult for those experiencing them, this condition should also not be surprising, based on what God has revealed about the pervasiveness of sin's disordering influence.

There are many things that could be said about the always fallible ways in which our culture, and every culture, defines true masculinity or true femininity. But as helpful as it would be to explore that topic, we first need to hear from God. The Hebrew and Christian Scriptures address these same issues (i.e., homosexuality, gender confusion) in a number of places (Leviticus 20:13; Deuteronomy 22:5; Romans 1:26, 27; I Corinthians 6:9, 10; I Timothy 1:8-11). While some of the specifics in these passages can be difficult to parse because of our cultural distance, understood in light of what God has revealed about the reality of our duality and the centrality of the "one flesh" union, we shouldn't be surprised by the serious and strong tone of these texts (e.g., that such behaviors are labeled "sin"). Whether we struggle personally with these kinds of feelings/desires, or know someone who does, it's important to remember that God cares. Again, we may not choose the struggles we experience, but we are able to choose our response. Thus, God is calling us to carefully consider every sexual urge in light of what he's revealed about sex, through both the 'book' of Nature (sound biology) and the book of Scripture (sound theology). Will we choose to live in light of the Designer's design, or contrary to those revelations, following the path of sin and self?

Summing It Up

Perspective and practice. What does it look like when our practice is shaped by God's perspective? Paul sums things up well in I Thessalonians 4:3-5...

> *For this is the will of God, your sanctification: that you abstain from sexual immorality; that each one of you know how to control his own body in holiness and honor, not in the passion of lust...*

So we could say that an incomparably good God's *self-revelation* in Scripture brings us to a place of *self-awareness* in terms of our compromised condition, that should lead to a life of *self-control* when it comes to our sexual urges. To be clear, pleasure is a gift from God. But when we choose "to enjoy the fleeting pleasures of sin" (Hebrews 11:25) over and against the lasting pleasure of knowing and serving an everlasting God, we forfeit the opportunity to experience pleasure as its (and our) Creator intended.

Now at this point, in light of this chapter, one of any number of words might be at the forefront of your mind. For some it might be "interesting" or "helpful". But for others, it might be "insensitive" or "intolerant". Still others might be thinking something like "unrealistic" or "unattainable". Or maybe, instead, you're wrestling with words like "ashamed", or "hopeless", or "confused". Whatever you're presently thinking and feeling, I want to encourage you to keep reading. Please. In the next chapter, the final chapter of this book, there is good news... very good news. If what you believe about sex is fueled by love, by giving love and receiving love, you'll definitely want to keep reading.

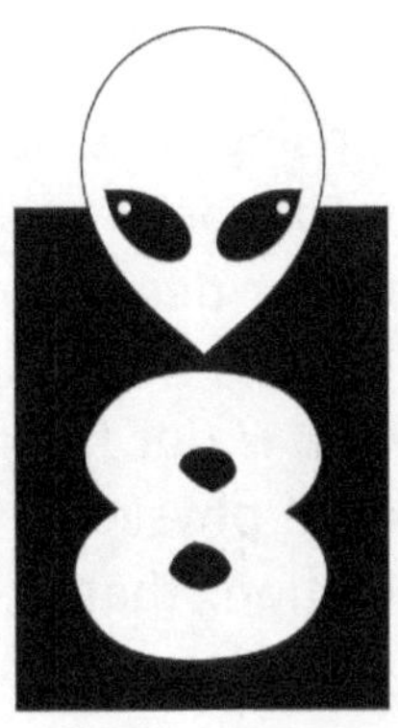

Looking Up

Strangely, you're just now hearing the birds, feeling the breeze, and smelling the smells of that grassy meadow. You're just now getting your bearings. How long have you been standing here, staring into the sky? You're not sure. But it's been a while since the alien spacecraft zoomed out of sight. Losing track of time is understandable when it comes to processing a 'close encounter' like the one we experienced. But don't go, not yet. Let's stay. Let's keep looking up. No, not for an extraterrestrial encore. Let's keep looking above us, to the One who is above all things.

In considering what God has revealed in sacred Scripture about sex, we were looking for help from beyond the stars; in fact, from the One who made the stars. But thankfully, his revelation encompasses far more than sexuality. Life is more than just satisfying our sexual appetites, right? Think about it: aren't there far deeper appetites driving our sexual desires?

Sex as Salvation

It shouldn't be surprising that our physical longings are driven by even deeper longings. For example, more powerful than our desire for a particular body is our desire to belong. More gripping than our hunger for stimulation is our hunger for affirmation. Wanting to be wanted physically so often betrays a deep need for validation, that is, confirmation that we are someone *worth* wanting. As with food, finances, fame, and so many other things (which may or may not begin with the letter "f"), sex is often used as a tool to meet some deeper need: to distract, to medicate, to escape from a painful reality; to feel needed, to feel pretty, to feel in control, to feel loved, to feel something... anything.

Did you know God is the creator of both your physical and emotional longings? He designed us to crave connection. He made us with an appetite for acceptance. He put within us a hunger for both pleasure and purpose. Above all, he created us to give love and receive love. But wonderfully, he put these longings in you so that, ultimately, you might be satisfied in him. You were made to love so that you might love God above everything and everyone else. You were given a longing for love so that your heart might be quenched by the fullness of his lavish, never-failing, never-ending love.

But God also made us for one another. And so he designed things like marriage, sex, and the family as important mechanisms to meet our 'hard-wired' longings for human connection, companionship, and community. Connection, companionship, and community can certainly be found in many other places, but marriage and the home were designed to be the *first* place; to be foundational.

But as we've already seen, our sin is a disordering and destructive influence when it comes to God's design. What exactly does that mean? It means that since each of us has turned away from God (living *me-centered* rather than *God-centered* lives), we wrongly look for that ultimate belonging, acceptance, validation, security, pleasure, purpose, and love in other people and other things. Thus we turn secondary things into primary things. That means we turn to things like sex in order to find what only God can give us, and in so doing, turn sex into something it was never meant to be.

The Bad News About Sex

But that leads us to some very bad news. Tragically, there's a lot of bad news that flows from our distortion of God's design: the broken heart of a jilted teen, the spread of sexually transmitted diseases, the betrayal of adultery, the objectification of women, sexual harassment, broken homes, prostitution, trafficking, rape, molestation, abortion. And the list could go on. But if you can believe it, there is something far worse when it comes to our misdirected urges and their consequences. Listen to the entirety of chapter 13, verse 4, of the book of Hebrews...

Let marriage be held in honor among all, and let the marriage bed be undefiled, for God will judge the sexually immoral and adulterous.

If sex is the sacred creation of the Master Artist, then our distortions of his design are not simply regrettable. They are reprehensible. If God is the center of all things, and absolute right and wrong flow directly from his character, then all of our sexual choices are moral choices. And as such, they will either align with or deviate from his good, loving, life-producing design. When they do deviate, they ultimately deviate for one, fundamental reason: *the autonomy of the self*. Therefore our rejection of God's good design (in all things) is a rejection of God as God. It is rebellion.

But there is only one God. There can only be one God. Therefore, God cannot and will not endure rivals. Because he is good, he is just. And because he is just, he will judge us and our distortions... *for God will judge the sexually immoral and adulterous*. That warning is given to both the unmarried and the married. All of us are accountable, not simply in the area of sexual choices, but in every area. No, we will not be judged for the ways we're tempted. God understands our weaknesses. But we will be judged for every compromise, every act of surrender; choosing what we desire over and against what God desires. While this may be good news for the cause of ultimate justice, it is bad news for sinners like us.

Grace Saves the Day

So God, the Judge (yep, that's a capital "J") of all judges, rightly hands down an *indictment* against rebels like us. And yet, amazingly, he also issues an *invitation*. No, not an invitation to get what we deserve. Shockingly, it's an invitation to get exactly the opposite of what we deserve. The Apostle Paul explained this strange but wonderful thing called "grace" throughout his writings, including Ephesians 2:1-10. Let me break that passage into three parts and provide a few comments after each part. Listen carefully to the incredible words in 2:1-3:

> *And you were dead in the trespasses and sins in which you once walked, following the course of this world, following the prince of the power of the air, the spirit that is now at work in the sons of disobedience—among whom we all once lived in the passions of our flesh, carrying out the desires of the body and the mind, and were by nature children of wrath, like the rest of mankind.*

"By nature" we are "children of wrath". That means something deep inside us is bent, bent toward self. But *me-centeredness* in a *God-centered* universe can only bring down the "wrath" of our just Judge (the result being eternal suffering under God's just sentence). Being "dead" to God, we live only for ourselves. As we've discussed, that means a life guided by "the passions of our flesh" and "the desires of the body and the mind". There are no exceptions ("we all") when it comes to those "following the course of this world".

> *But God, being rich in mercy, because of the great love with which he loved us, even when we were dead in our trespasses, made us alive together with Christ—by grace you have been saved—and raised us up with him and seated us with him in the heavenly places in Christ Jesus, so that in the coming ages he might show the immeasurable riches of his grace in kindness toward us in Christ Jesus.*

These verses (2:4-7) reveal that the love for which we're ultimately made is available to us today. Yes, today! Through his incomparable love, God can make us "alive together with Christ". That means just as Jesus was raised to life after his death on a Roman cross, we too can be raised, to a new spiritual life in this world, and a new (free of defects) bodily life in the world to come. How is this possible when we are "dead in our trespasses " (i.e., sins)? Grace! Grace is God's undeserved kindness, the gift of unearned favor. Grace is God giving us exactly the opposite of what we deserve. Paul tells his readers, "by grace you have been saved" from a wrath-filled, God-less eternity.

But what about our "trespasses"? Paul reminded his readers at the beginning of this letter that in Jesus "we have redemption through his blood, the forgiveness of our trespasses, according to the riches of his grace..." (1:7). Because Jesus shed his blood, giving his life on that cross to accept the just penalty our sins deserve, we can now know "forgiveness". "Redemption" means Jesus paid our debt, a debt he did not owe, but one he knew we could not pay. A third set of verses from Ephesians 2, verses 8-10, tells us more about God's grace...

> *For by grace you have been saved through faith. And this is not your own doing; it is the gift of God, not a result of works, so that no one may boast. For we are his workmanship, created in Christ Jesus for good works, which God prepared beforehand, that we should walk in them.*

"Grace" has nothing to do with "your own doing". God's gift of life is "not a result of works" we can list on a religious résumé. Thankfully, grace is disconnected from what we actually deserve for our actual works. What then can we do? All we can do is believe Jesus did it all. That's what it means to be "saved through faith". When we turn to Christ and trust Christ as our only hope, forgiveness and freedom are ours. Freedom? Yes, freedom to love God, and be loved by God. Mercifully, God sets us free from our *me-centered* shackles. By his divine power, if we are new by grace, "we are his workmanship", carefully crafted and purposely powered to live a new kind of life, one marked by "good works"; the overflow of a new, God-centered heart.

Good News for the Needy

That stunning message of grace for rebels, of forgiveness for sinners, of love for lost people like us, is what the New Testament calls the *gospel*. It's a word that simply means, "good news". And when it comes to sexuality in this straying and struggling world, it is good news indeed. In fact, it's the best news ever. Here's how. This message about Jesus, this gospel of grace is...

Good news for the loveless. Our world often struggles with the distinction between *love* and *lust*. For example, we strangely describe sexual intercourse, even between strangers, as 'making love'. Or think about a teenage girl who gives in to her boyfriend's lust, hoping to find love instead. Or what about a man working his way through a string of 'lovers', and yet losing his way in a fog of loneliness. As we've learned, all of us were made for connection. But a physical connection like sex cannot give us the spiritual connection for which we're ultimately hungry, for the higher love for which we were made. But wonderfully, the grace of God in Jesus makes this very thing possible.

Good news for the rudderless. In light of sin's disordering influence, understanding our sexual urges in a sexually confused world is no easy task. Which voice are we to believe, and why? Who truly cares? When we move past caricatures and misinformation about this message, the good news about Jesus should be our *true north*. It alone reveals both the affection and authority for which we long. In embracing Jesus by faith we discover not only God's loving hand, but also his leading hand. God places in us a desire to become like the One who became like us; as was stated in an earlier chapter, "the One who stepped *inside* humanity from *outside* the world, in order to save the world." And this "word of the cross" (I Corinthians 1:18) leads us to all of God's words in Scripture. Because of our world and our hearts, we desperately need light. Wonderfully, the grace of God in Jesus makes this very thing possible.

Good news for the powerless. Maybe you are reading this book and you are hungry for the change God describes. Maybe you see the beauty and goodness of his design, but feel helpless to heed his words. Using words from the previous chapter, maybe you have been brought to a place of *self-awareness* in terms of your compromised condition, but feel far from *self-control* when it comes to your sexual urges. Well, be encouraged. The gospel is good news for the powerless. Writing to a young man named Timothy almost two thousand years ago, the Apostle Paul encouraged him in light of the fact that, through Jesus, "God gave us a spirit...of power and love and self-control." (II Timothy 1:7). While your inclinations may seem insurmountable, God is more powerful than your desires. Your weakness needs his strength. Wonderfully, the grace of God in Jesus makes this very thing possible.

Good news for the comfortless. Sexuality detached from God's design is a destructive force. Sadly, a system designed to produce life has robbed so many of the kind of life we desire for those we love. Instead of joy and peace, so many today are weighed down by fears or frustrations, by guilt or grief, by anger or anxiety, because of their own or someone else's sexual sin. There's the woman who was raped in college. There's the man who was molested as a child. There's the teen wrestling with shame after 'sexting' a classmate. There's the young woman grappling with her heart, after just trading sexual favors for a promotion at work. And the list could go on. But no matter the heaviness of the hurt or the grip of the guilt, in Jesus, God's love can bring comfort to the needy heart; the promise of his reassuring presence; the reality of his forgiveness and unconditional love. For some, such comfort seems almost too good to be true. But wonderfully, the grace of God in Jesus makes this very thing possible.

Good news for the hopeless. Sex is a fleeting pleasure. That doesn't make it a bad thing. But that does make it an inferior option when it comes to finding ultimate fulfillment. And yet so many today look to sexual pleasures to provide the lasting satisfaction only God can give. But sexual pleasures, like all healthy, earthly pleasures, were designed to point us to God's presence. As King David wrote several thousand years ago, "You make known to me the path of life; in your presence there is fullness of joy; at your right hand are pleasures forevermore." (Psalm 16:11)

Real hope, sustaining hope, empowering hope is not hope in the next sexual encounter or conquest. It is hope, even in the worst of times, in the power and promises of a faithful, good, and unstoppable God; hope "that for those who love God all things work together for good, for those who are called according to his purpose..." (Romans 8:28). It is hope in the promise that God "will sustain you to the end, guiltless in the day of our Lord Jesus Christ. God is faithful..." (I Corinthians 1:8–9). It is hope in the promised future described in Revelation 21:3, 4...

> *And I heard a loud voice from the throne saying, "Behold, the dwelling place of God is with man. He will dwell with them, and they will be his people, and God himself will be with them as their God. He will wipe away every tear from their eyes, and death shall be no more, neither shall there be mourning, nor crying, nor pain anymore, for the former things have passed away."*

In our sexual struggles, our concerns about connection, and our longings for love, we desperately need this kind of hope. Wonderfully, the grace of God in Jesus makes this very thing possible.

Pushing the Boundaries

As we close in on the end of this book, would you do something for me? Would you go back and look at the bullet-pointed questions on page 40? I'll wait here while you do.

All finished? Good. After having worked through the second half of this book, I hope the connection between the meaning of life and the meaning of sex is a little clearer. Did you see how the the gospel of God's grace, how the good news about Jesus Christ, answers those ultimate questions about life? And when my deeper, driving questions are answered in my Creator, I begin to seek his guidance in every area of my everyday life. And that includes my sexuality.

Do you personally have answers to those questions? How you think about sex and sexuality is an indicator of how you think about everything, that is, it's an expression of your *worldview* (you may recall we talked about your take on the world in chapter 5). Some worldviews have very few answers when it comes to those ultimate questions; heavy on skepticism and speculation, but very few answers. Other worldviews can provide answers to those questions, but they are often internally inconsistent, historically problematic, and/or don't always correspond to our everyday observations and common sense intuitions. But again, what about you? If someone asked you why you believe what you believe about sex and sexuality, how would you explain the 'roots' of your perspective?

At the end of the first part of this book, I described my 'bare bones' goal for every reader: that each person would... *explore, and then eventually embrace, an outlook on sex/sexuality that makes sense of both the clear function of our biology and the common flaws of our beliefs and behavior.*

Inspired by that statement, allow me, here at the end of the second half, to summarize a similar but broader goal. My hope is that you will walk away from Part Two of this book, that you will walk from this book as a whole, encouraged *to explore, and then eventually embrace, an outlook on life that truly makes sense of what the world is like, and what people are like (inside and out), in light of humanity's ultimate questions.*

My aim in this second half was simply to present a clear case for the Christian worldview (i.e., "an outlook on life" informed by the Jewish and Christian Scriptures), specifically, how that worldview helps us make sense of the functions, feelings, and yes, even the flaws of the human sexual system. If I've been able to clarify certain things in your mind, or even tie things together, I'm thankful. If I've been able to challenge you to live for something bigger than lust, and more sacred than self, I'm thankful. If I've been able to help you understand why your neighbor or coworker or family member thinks the way they do, I'm thankful. If I've been able to direct you to the comfort, healing, hope, grace, purpose, and love that only God can give, I'm thankful.

But if after finishing this book you find that you simply cannot agree with its arguments (or at least many of its arguments), then I'd ask you to do one more thing for me: please take some time to think about why. Are there good reasons to reject the ideas explained in this book? Well, as the author of the book, I don't think there are (if I believed there were, I would not have written this book in the first place—he said wryly, but playfully). But if there were good reasons, they would be based on a careful consideration of *what the world is [really] like, and what people are [really] like (inside and out), in light of humanity's ultimate questions.* Objections would be based on objectivity, at least to the best of one's ability. That's not to say feelings are irrelevant, or that personal preferences should be tossed out. But reasoning based mainly on one's feelings, experiences, wants, etc. should be questioned and considered in light of the shared assumptions, verifiable propositions, and common sense intuitions that underlie all of our daily interactions and decisions. Every single one of us needs and depends on regular 'course corrections' when it comes to our feelings, since at times, feelings can be poor indicators of what is true, or right, or helpful, or healthy in any given situation.

How might I sum up these final encouragements? In the words of the subheading of this section, don't be afraid to 'push the boundaries'. Some have felt, and many still feel, that pushing boundaries when it comes to sex is all about being *untethered* from traditional taboos and 'repressive' rules. But I would argue (as I've attempted to do in this book) that the real *sexual revolutionary* is the man or woman who resists the tyranny of self, who rebels against society's squishy subjectivity, and looks beyond (ultimately above) themselves for direction in light of our defects, disorders, and deviations. I would argue that real *sexual liberation* is freedom *from* our culture's sexual idolatry, and freedom *to* follow our Creator's path. But neither star-surfing aliens nor spiritual aliens can set us free in that way. Only the most influential individual in human history can do that; the man who died and rose again; the God who came from 'out there' to love us right here. Though it's borrowed from a bumper sticker, it's true nonetheless: in the end, *no matter the sexual question, the answer is "Jesus"*.